Rafael Yépez

Frequency of attempted self-harm and associated risk factors

Rafael Yépez

Frequency of attempted self-harm and associated risk factors

In patients from 7 to 13 years of age

Imprint

Any brand names and product names mentioned in this book are subject to trademark, brand or patent protection and are trademarks or registered trademarks of their respective holders. The use of brand names, product names, common names, trade names, product descriptions etc. even without a particular marking in this work is in no way to be construed to mean that such names may be regarded as unrestricted in respect of trademark and brand protection legislation and could thus be used by anyone.

Cover image: www.ingimage.com

This book is a translation from the original published under ISBN 978-613-9-00059-3.

Publisher:
Sciencia Scripts
is a trademark of
Dodo Books Indian Ocean Ltd. and OmniScriptum S.R.L publishing group

120 High Road, East Finchley, London, N2 9ED, United Kingdom
Str. Armeneasca 28/1, office 1, Chisinau MD-2012, Republic of Moldova, Europe
Printed at: see last page
ISBN: 978-620-7-94316-6

Copyright © Rafael Yépez
Copyright © 2024 Dodo Books Indian Ocean Ltd. and OmniScriptum S.R.L publishing group

Contents

I dedicate this work mainly to God, for giving me life and allowing me to reach this important moment in my professional training.

To my mother, for being the most important pillar and for always showing me her unconditional love and support, always studying late and taking care of all my meals.

To my uncle who stayed up many early mornings and went out no matter what the weather was like to help me fulfil my obligations.

To my grandparents for their unconditional support and for being proud to see me achieve my goals, especially my beautiful old lady who left me half way through, but I know she is happy to see me achieve another goal.

To the one who has put up with me day after day during these three years, filling me with patience in every episode of stress and joy, always giving me her unconditional support and trying to do the best for me, Ana María.

To my house of studies, UCLA - HUPAZ for allowing me to train with the best, temporarily becoming my second home, providing me with knowledge and experiences.

To my colleagues and friends from graduate school and team 6, who together with our eternal bosses, also contributed to my training.

To my brothers in life, Yurhlio, Elías and Horacio, with the three of them as my support the burdens became more bearable, thank you for your sincere support. To my blood brothers and sisters for always being there for me, especially my black one. To my dad for being proud of my achievements.

To each of my teachers, who, being of such different characters, are capable of working together to make everything work correctly, especially to Pelón (Dr Aranguren), an open book who teaches you word by word; to Dr Carnevale, Dr Santana, Dr Palacios, Dr Ferrer, Dr Rivas, Dr Uzcátegui, Dr Méndez, Dr Pacheco and Dr Rubio.

To my internship graduates and the on-call team, who with a lot of patience are able to put up with everything that happens to us on each shift and also took care of making me gain kilo by kilo with each meal, especially Yessica, Adriana, Migdalia and Dayana, my blacks.

And last but not least to the postgraduate mother that life gave me, a woman so full of virtues that she is capable of overshadowing all the bad things that surround us, Thank you Sibeida Bracho, the stainless steel cover has already melted!!!!.

SUMMARY

Autolysis is the act by which a person intentionally causes his or her own death. The aim of this research study was to determine the frequency of attempted self-harm and the associated risk factors in patients aged 7 to 13 years admitted to the Emergency Department of the Servicio Desconcentrado Hospital Universitario Pediátrico Dr. Agustín Zubillaga, during the period January 2017 to June 2022. A cross-sectional descriptive study was conducted, whose population consisted of patients aged 7 to 13 years, 11 months and 29 days, with a diagnosis of attempted autolysis, the sample was a non-probabilistic and intentional census sample adjusted to the selection criteria, then the data were recorded in an instrument developed for this purpose and applied through the review of medical records as a secondary source, the results were presented in tables or graphs and statistical analysis was performed using computerised statistical packages such as the Statistical Package for Social Sciences (SPSS), version 25.0 for calculations. Thus, analysing each of the responses, it is concluded that: Attempted self-harm comprised 51% aged 13 -15 years, of which 63% represented the female gender; the methods were 78% substance ingestion, 19% Hanging and 3% other; 6% died, 3% with sequelae, 61% graffar IV, 92% in schooling, 53% an absent father, 28% previous attempt, 50% due to discussion with a relative mostly with the mother, which allowed conclusions and recommendations to be drawn respectively.

Keywords: autolysis, risk factors, patients.

INTRODUCTION

The World Health Organisation (WHO 2020) records that some 800,000 people commit suicide each year, representing an estimated rate of 11.4 deaths per 100,000 inhabitants. Deaths by self-harm are the second leading cause of death among young people aged 15-29. Among the most common factors are family problems such as situations of physical and verbal violence, sexual abuse, school problems, both in relation to low grades, as well as rejection by the peer group which, in some cases, turns into bullying through teasing, discrimination and aggression.

For its part, the National Institute of Statistics and Census cited in Gerstner, (2018) mentions that suicide in Ecuador has increased, in the last two decades almost 300 young people and adolescents aged 10-24 years took their own lives annually. Suicide is a complex and multifactorial public health problem, so health promotion strategies in the country should be designed to reach the majority of the population in order to minimise the risk of suicide by removing barriers to care and implementing health policies with current records and thus reduce deaths by self-harm.

Likewise, child suicide, understood as that which occurs before the age of 14, is very uncommon because there is hardly any awareness of death and its implications, "....within those ages it is not common, because for suicide to be considered as such, there must be an explicit desire for death, in which the child must be aware of what death is, bearing in mind that these are concepts formed between the ages of 9 and 14", according to José Luis Pedreira, former president of the Child Psychiatry section of the Spanish Association of Paediatrics and psychiatrist at the Niño Jesús Hospital in Madrid, Spain.

With this in mind, there are many factors that may increase the risk of suicide in adolescents, as they may feel suicidal due to certain life circumstances such as: having a psychiatric disorder such as depression, an anxiety disorder, bipolar disorder or oppositional defiant disorder, family history of mood disorder, suicidality or suicidal behaviour, history of physical or sexual abuse, or exposure to violence or bullying, a substance use disorder, access to means such as firearms or medication, exposure to the suicide of a family member or friend, a loss or conflict involving close friends or family members, physical or medical problems such as puberty-related changes or chronic illness, children who have attempted suicide in the past are also at increased risk. (Kennebeck S, et al 2021)

In the United States, suicide attempts are more frequent in adolescent girls than in boys, but boys are more likely to die by suicide. It is important to consider that adolescents do not have the life experience to know that these things will be temporary, that they will get over them, it is inferred that they might think they would rather be dead than feel that way at that moment, and persistent misunderstandings about suicide can also prevent adolescents from getting the help they need. (Asarnow, Hughes, Babeva, Sugar 2017).

Some of the warning signs of an adolescent thinking about suicide are talking about wanting to die, feeling desperate, being trapped or being in unbearable pain. This is why this study is so important to try to protect people's integrity, which is a right guaranteed by the state. In these conditions, the present study aims to determine the frequency of attempted self-harm and the associated risk factors in patients between 7 and 13 years of age who are admitted to the emergency department of the deconcentrated service of the University Paediatric Hospital Dr. Agustín Zubillaga during the period of January to December of the same year. Agustín Zubillaga during the period January 2017 to June 2022, through a cross-sectional descriptive field study, since an interdisciplinary team trained in the management of patients for this pathology should be available to ensure optimal care in patient care. Therefore, this study is structured as follows:

Chapter I deals with the problems posed, the general and specific objectives and the justification for the study.

Chapter II refers to the background of research related to the topic under study and describes the theoretical and legal bases that support the research. The variables are also operationalised.

In Chapter III, the methodological framework is described in accordance with the type of research, population and sample, data collection technique, and the procedure for the development of the research.

Chapter IV describes the results and discussion and Chapter V the conclusions and recommendations. Finally, bibliographical references and annexes are included.

CHAPTER I

THE PROBLEM
Problem Statement

Adolescence is a transcendental and critical stage for human development, due to the series of physiological, psychological and interpersonal changes it entails. These changes make the adolescent vulnerable, as an identity crisis arises that confronts them with themselves, family demands and society, producing great anxiety, feelings that, on occasions, adolescents are unable to cope with, due to different factors, including their personality characteristics, daily stress and the absence of social and family support networks, factors that favour the presence of emotional distress in adolescents, which can lead to risky behaviour, such as: drug use and suicide attempts, which compromise their physical and psychological integrity.

This is why self-harm is considered a public health problem, which ranks among the leading causes of premature death and accounts for 1.4% of the global burden of disease in disability-adjusted life years. Completed suicide is the leading cause of external death in many countries around the world and one of the leading causes of death in adolescents and people of productive age.

Risk factors associated with attempted self-harm in children are also related to family dysfunction, the presence of family history and/or parents with self-harm attempts, and family conflicts leading to poor parent-child relationships. McKeown and collaborators (1998) attempted to define the predisposing factors for suicidal behaviour in a population of North American adolescents, who were followed up for one year, showing that family cohesion was an evident protective factor. In Chile, attempted suicide in children and adolescents has been studied in several regions of the country. In 1983, a review of 22 children admitted for attempted suicide at the Dr. Exequiel González Cortés Children's Hospital in Santiago showed that the relevant conditions associated with suicidal behaviour were a poor parent-child relationship, poor intrafamily communication and parental overprotection.

Similarly, dealing with the subject of suicide is complicated by the fact that many factors are involved. It should be borne in mind that in Spain, in the last recorded year, there were a total of 3,941 cases, of which the number of suicides is higher in males than in females, with an average of 2.65 per 100,000 inhabitants, in the young population between 15-19 years of age. The Canary Islands have the highest percentage of suicides in Spain, according to the National Institute of Statistics (INE), with a total of 208 deaths by suicide, 1.28%, which is well ahead of the second place, the Balearic Islands. Due to the large increase in voluntary drug poisoning (VMI), with a self-inflicted suicide attempt (SA), especially in the last two years, specifically related to the appearance of the COVID-19 pandemic, where the number of this type of patients is increasing, and a common action guide is necessary.

Since the start of the pandemic, hospitals in the United States have seen more mental health emergencies among children; between March and October 2020, the percentage of emergency department visits for children with mental health emergencies increased by 24% for children aged 5-11 years and 31% for children aged 12-17 years. There was also an increase of more than 50% in emergency department visits for suspected suicide attempts among girls aged 12-17 years in early 2021 compared to the same period in 2019. The COVID-19 pandemic has taken a heavy toll on children's mental health, as young people continue to face physical isolation, constant uncertainty, fear and pain. In addition, many young people have been affected by the loss of a loved one, with recent data showing that more than 140,000 US children have experienced the death of a primary or secondary caregiver during the COVID-19 pandemic.

In this sense, considering the precarious situation of the problem, it is imperative to carry out actions for its prevention. In fact, the Pan American Health Organization 2014 (PAHO) has already called on the different countries of the world to include suicide prevention in their health "agendas". Among the actions that can be implemented are training, information, awareness-raising and sensitisation of society in general, and of psychology professionals in particular. Suicidal behaviour prevention strategies can also be implemented in social, health and/or educational contexts, to name but a few.

Indeed, prevention measures in the field of suicide have shown their effectiveness, making it clear that suicide is preventable. One form of prevention is the early detection and identification of a possible case of suicide risk or screening of participants in samples of the general population who may be at risk. Once a potential case has been detected and identified, evidence-based prophylactic treatments could be implemented, with the usual benefits on multiple levels; let's be clear, the earlier it is detected and identified, and the more effective the intervention, the better.

Bearing this in mind, it is worrying that, knowing this reality, there is little evidence of intervention for early identification in primary care services in health centres, which would minimise admissions to the emergency department; in fact, if there were better treatment in the preventive area, the number of attempts at self-harm and appearances in the emergency department would be considerably reduced. There is also a lack of protocols for multidisciplinary action in these cases, which would help to develop strategies and treatments to act on these patients and their environment, and the decentralised service of the Dr. Agustín Zubillaga University Paediatric Hospital does not escape from this reality. For this reason, this field, descriptive, cross-sectional research will be carried out with the aim of determining the frequency of attempted self-harm and the associated risk factors in patients aged 7 to 13 years who are admitted to the emergency department of the Dr. Agustín Zubillaga University Paediatric Hospital during the period January 2017 to June 2022.

Taking into account the above, considering that to date in the aforementioned hospital there has been common evidence of young people attempting self-harm, an alarming situation due to its consequences, the following question arises: What is the frequency of self-harm and the associated risk factors in young people aged 7 to 13 years at the Servicio Desconcentrado Hospital Universitario Pediátrico Dr. Agustín Zubillaga during the period January 2017 to June 2022?

Research Objectives

General Objective

To determine the frequency of attempted autolysis and associated risk factors in patients aged 7 to 13 years admitted to the emergency department of the Dr. Agustín Zubillaga University Paediatric Hospital during the period January 2017 to June 2022.

Specific Objectives

1   To identify the socio-demographic characteristics of patients aged 7 to 13 years admitted for attempted self-harm.

2   To describe the clinical characteristics of patients aged 7 to 13 years admitted for attempted self-harm.

3   To recognise the risk factors of patients aged 7 to 13 years admitted for attempted self-harm.

4   To detail the physical sequelae resulting from attempted self-harm in patients aged 7 to 13 years admitted for this pathology.

5   To identify the mechanisms of attempted autolysis in patients aged 7 to 13 years admitted for this pathology.

6   To indicate the frequency of death in patients aged 7 to 13 years admitted for attempted self-harm.

Justification and Importance

The development of this study is important from a theoretical point of view, as it allowed a literature review to be carried out and updated knowledge to be acquired by the medical team in charge of its development, with reference to self-harm in young people. Furthermore, it is known that, from a practical point of view, the development of a responsible attitude on the part of parents by going to care centres from the beginning of the manifestations of suicidal behaviour in search of help can be avoided, which is precisely where the social relevance of the study lies.

In this study, the possibility of relating attempts at self-harm and their increase in recent years to the current pandemic situation was considered, as a possible effect of all the isolation and distancing measures that have led to less contact between families, especially in those where the predictors (history of personal and family self-harm) are exacerbated compared to families where there is no history of self-harm.

From the scientific point of view, the present research arose from the need to strengthen the knowledge of the health team, to know the current characteristics of autolysis in young people, allowing the updating of information on the subject of study in the Immediate Medical Attention Service of the Servicio de Atención Médica Inmediata del Servicio Desconcentrado Hospital Universitario Pediátrico Dr. Agustín Zubillaga, likewise, we do not rule out the possibility that methodologically it could serve to initiate other research on the subject from other perspectives.

From a social and educational point of view, prevention through educational guidance on child care given to mothers aims to reduce morbidity and mortality in children, which is why education must be provided in a comprehensive manner, considering each of the factors that relate to mothers and children, i.e. considering them in their biopsychosocial environment.

Similarly, from a medical and public health perspective, it is essential that medical staff and the health team in general comply with and perfect preventive strategies, as this is one of their main duties towards the user, family and community. This greatly benefits the child by maintaining a better quality of life, while at the same time optimising health care resources and, in particular, providing stability and family wellbeing.

CHAPTER II

THEORETICAL FRAMEWORK

In this research context, the theories that guide the research are set out, in order to condition the scientific information that exists on the variables to be studied, allowing knowledge to be improved and leading to the meaning that is to be given to the study. For his part, Arias (2014) argues that the theoretical framework "expresses the general theoretical propositions, specific theories, postulates, assumptions, categories and concepts that are to serve as a reference to order the mass of facts concerning the problem that are the subject of study and research" (p.100). The theoretical framework of this research is broken down from the background, the theoretical bases, the legal bases and the system of variables.

Tamayo and Tamayo (2020) argue that the background "tries to make a conceptual synthesis of the research, in order to determine the methodological approach of the research". (p. 54), the theoretical framework and the background of the research seek to highlight the similarity that exists between research carried out in previous years, conserving the same variable under study, in this case, autolysis in young people, which will serve as support for the development of this work.

There is some research on the topic of the study, which evaluates variables similar to the objective of the study. The most relevant publications are listed below.

According to Arencibia (2022) who conducted a study entitled attempted self-harm by intoxication in young people in the Canary Islands: emergency department of the University Hospital Complex of the Canary Islands; taking this into account, the World Health Organisation (WHO) defines mental health as the state of well-being of an individual, in which he or she is able to cope with the obstacles of everyday life, work effectively and contribute to his or her community. The present study was conducted at the Complejo Universitario de Canarias (CHUC) in Tenerife, Canary Islands, specifically from November 2021 to December 2021. This study aims to identify the frequency of patients admitted with a diagnosis of suicide attempt due to drug intoxication, as well as to determine the determining factors of this situation, and which method has been used. The relevance of this study is due to the high number of young patients with psychiatric problems and attempted self-harm received by the Emergency Department of the CHUC, which makes a protocol for this type of case indispensable. It is clearly visible that we are dealing with a major public health problem, the rise of which has greatly increased since COVID-19, making it necessary to employ measures of action to reduce suicide attempts in the young population and, therefore, mortality in this sector of the population.

In this regard, mention should be made of the work carried out by Vega (2021), who carried out a study entitled deaths by autolysis at the Forensic Science Research Centre in Loja-Ecuador, in which he states: autolysis constitutes a very important public health problem, but to a large extent preventable, visualised as an escape from a problem or a crisis that produces intense suffering, and that is why it is important to communicate to the public through current records in order to be able to initiate prevention plans. In this research we determined the main mechanism of autolysis, identified the most susceptible sex and age group, as well as the main predisposing factors related to deaths by autolysis registered at the Forensic Science Research Centre in the periods 2016 to 2019, which were known through the forensic medical report.

A descriptive, retrospective study was carried out, in which the population included deceased citizens who had lived in the provinces of Loja and Zamora Chinchipe; a total of 134 cases were obtained; hanging was determined to be the most common mechanism used; the most affected sex was male; the most prevalent age groups were those aged between 14 and 20 years, and the predisposing factors that led to this decision were love break-ups and depression.

Similarly, Fonseca (2020) carried out a study entitled Assessment of suicidal behaviour in adolescents: about the Paykel Suicide Scale. Suicidal behaviour is a socio-health problem worldwide; however, in the context of Spanish psychology, there are few measurement instruments that have been properly validated and assessed in representative samples of the adolescent population. Therefore, the purpose of this paper is to present the Paykel Suicide Scale as a tool for the assessment of suicidal behaviour in young Spaniards. First, a brief conceptual delimitation of suicidal behaviour, epidemiological data, psychological models and risk and protective factors are mentioned. Secondly, the assessment of suicidal behaviour is addressed as a central axis in the detection, identification, prevention and intervention, as well as in the understanding of this phenomenon. Thirdly, the Paykel Suicide Scale is introduced, with its psychometric properties and, specifically, its assessment in Spanish adolescents.

Finally, it is concluded by way of recapitulation: The Paykel Scale appears to be a brief, simple, useful and useful measurement instrument with adequate psychometric properties for the assessment and/or screening of suicidal behaviour in adolescents. It can be used in general mental health assessment or psychopathological screening, as well as in educational, health and/or social contexts. It is crucial that the psychology professional has adequate tools for the assessment of suicidal behaviour in order to make informed decisions and optimise the management of educational and social-health resources.

Theoretical basis

Suicide

According to Villamar (2015), the WHO defines suicide as "an act with lethal consequences, intentionally initiated and carried out by the individual, knowing or expecting its lethal outcome and through which he or she intends to obtain the desired changes". In order to operationalise the concepts and terminology around suicide, it is important to make a distinction between:

- Suicidal behaviour: group of behaviours with or without fatal outcome, including suicide attempt or suicide.
- Suicidal ideation: thoughts that can range from ideas that life is not worth living, to intense self-harming preoccupations or well-structured plans about how to die.
- Suicide: intentional and self-directed act resulting in death.
- Suicide attempt: a self-directed, non-fatal, potentially harmful act that seeks death.

Epidemiology

According to WHO estimates, one of the most worrying data worldwide is the increase in suicide rates among young people (15-29 years), making it one of the three most frequent causes of death in this age group. Most national and international studies have highlighted this increase at young ages, especially in males. Worldwide, suicidal ideation and non-suicidal self-harm are a very frequent reason for consultation in paediatric, primary care and emergency departments. It is estimated that approximately 5 out of every 100 000 adolescents commit suicide each year; 3-6% make a suicide attempt during their lifetime, 30% have suicidal ideation, and 18% cause self-harm without lethal intent (cuts, scratches, burns, poisoning, among others) (Villamar ob.cit).

According to a study published in the journal The Lancet, 1 in 12 children between the ages of 9 and 10 reported having had suicidal thoughts, but little is said about this, which is why Álvaro Jiménez, an academic at the Faculty of Psychology at the UDP and researcher at the Millennium Nucleus for Improving the Mental Health of Adolescents and Young People (Imhay), says "regarding child suicide, it is difficult to study it because statistically there are few cases to draw the right conclusions"; It is believed that this taboo has been installed because there is a false conception that holds that schoolchildren, as part of their cognitive development, do not think about these issues, "and if they do, they communicate it very little, in comparison with adolescents". It is important to remember that between the ages of 8 and 9, death begins to be symbolised as a natural and irreversible phenomenon, so at that age it is essential to be alert to certain signs, especially because child suicide is associated with a type of behaviour that is more impulsive than in other age groups.

In Ecuador, between 2001 and 2014, 4855 deaths by suicide of adolescents and young people were registered, most of them males aged 15 to 24 years old. In 2017, according to data from the National Directorate of Crimes against Life, Violent Deaths, Disappearances, Extortion and Kidnappings (DINASED), suicide has become the leading cause of death in adolescents, the rate was 6.4 per 100 000 adolescents between 10 and 17 years of age. In Cuenca, in 2019, a descriptive cross-sectional correlational study was conducted in students of the "Unidad Educativa Dora Beatriz Canelos", 38 cases (29.01%) with suicidal behaviour were found. The most frequent age was 15-18 years (16.79%), and the sex with the greatest predisposition was male (15.27%). It also points out that every year in Ecuador, 352.6 people die from unspecified events. These events could be a source of hidden suicides, of which men represent 76.39% (Aucapiña 2019).

According to Nixon et al, (2008) mentions that non-suicidal self-harm occurs most frequently between the ages of 11 and 15 years (73%). Similarly, Argota et al, (2014), indicate that non-suicidal self-harm occurred more frequently in the female sex, representing 74.5%, and in the 15-19 age group, 63.4%. According to studies reviewed up to 2018, suicidal behaviour is more frequent in the female population (68%), with an age of onset ranging from 13 to 15 years.

Risk Factors

Several risk factors related to suicidal and non-suicidal self-harming behaviours have been described in the literature and will be detailed below (Daniel, et al. 2017).

1. Individual factors: depression, previous suicide attempt, gender, age, substance abuse.

2. Family factors: family functionality, presence of parental migration, stressful life events, social network.

3. Other factors: Being a victim of physical, sexual or psychological violence, peer harassment.

4. Economic income: the risk of suicide is doubled among young people with socio-economic status, economic conflict has been reported to increase the risk of suicidal behaviour twice, and earning less than the unified minimum wage has a high statistical significance for committing non-suicidal self-harm.

5. Family Functionality: The family constitutes the individual's first support network, which is why it is conceived as having a protective function in the face of the stresses of everyday life; conflicts, violence and negative relationships between family members are closely related to suicidal behaviour; the presence of non-suicidal self-harm, on the other hand, indicates that adolescents from dysfunctional families are 4 times more at risk of non-suicidal self-harm.

6. Parental migration: Parental migration leads to family disintegration, resulting in the loss of affective ties, which places the adolescent in a highly vulnerable situation, i.e. there is an increased risk that his or her physical and emotional integrity will be harmed.

7. Belonging to a social group: Belonging to a social group becomes a necessity; permanent and prolonged contact with a social group can act as a protective factor when the adolescent manages to identify with and belong to this group, finding affective links.

8. Depression: It is a mood disorder, which generates alterations in mood and affects their relationship with other people, being a risk factor for the health of adolescents, since depression and suicidal thoughts are related according to several studies, however, there is not always an early detection and mood swings, melancholy and affective lability in adolescents are usually considered as normal. People affected by depression are 20 times more likely to be at risk of suicide than the average population.

9. Use of psychoactive substances: The use of psychoactive substances has been strongly associated with suicidal risk, with approximately one third of men and one fifth of women who attempt suicide abusing alcohol, cigarettes or other substances that alter the nervous system.

10. Victims of violence (physical, sexual and psychological): The abuse, whether physical or verbal, is justified by parents as a way of educating, with women being the main victims, this

technique has been maintained throughout time, parents believe that this is the only way to maintain a balance in the family, however, this can lead to serious consequences and adolescents, feeling that they are not loved, may even have the desire to end their lives. Studies show that adolescents who suffer physical or psychological violence are twice as likely to be suicidal and are statistically associated with self-harm. Children subjected to physical and sexual violence have a high incidence of suicidal behaviour.

Legal Basis

The present study is based from the legal point of view on the Constitution of the Bolivarian Republic of Venezuela (1999) in Chapter V. On Social Rights and Families, where Article 83 states that health is a fundamental right, and the State has the obligation to guarantee it as part of the right to life. Therefore, it must promote and develop policies that lead to an improvement in the quality of life, collective well-being and access to services.

Likewise, Article 84 mentions that the right to health is guaranteed through the creation of a national public health system that is free, universal, comprehensive, equitable and supportive, which gives priority to health promotion and disease prevention, guaranteeing timely treatment and quality rehabilitation.

Similarly, the Organic Law on Social Security (2002) in Article 18, paragraph one, ratifies the above, since the State must promote the health of the entire population in a universal and equitable manner, which must include protection and education for health and quality of life, the prevention of diseases and accidents, the restoration of health and rehabilitation; timely, adequate and of high quality.

On the other hand, the Law on the Practice of Medicine (2011) Title III, Chapter II Research on Human Subjects cites in Article 93 that "Clinical research is only permissible when conducted and supervised by scientifically qualified persons". While article 97 states that the person must be well informed of everything related to the research and give consent to participate, it also states that in case of legal or physical incapacity, consent must be obtained in writing from the patient's legal representative and, in the absence of the latter, from the patient's closest responsible family member.

The above shows that this research work is in line with the legal framework in force in the Bolivarian Republic of Venezuela. There are no constitutional limitations or national, regional or local laws that restrict this type of research; on the contrary, there is a legal and regulatory framework that supports the importance of carrying out this study.

CHAPTER III

METHODOLOGICAL FRAMEWORK

Type of research

Non-experimental research of a descriptive and cross-sectional nature was carried out. It is non-experimental, as Palella and Martins (2012) define it as that which is carried out without deliberately manipulating any variable, observing the facts as they are presented in their real context and at a given time or not, in order to then analyse them, therefore, in this design a specific situation is not constructed, but rather those that exist are observed.

On the other hand, it is considered descriptive because, according to the author Arias (2006), this type of study consists of the characterisation of a fact, phenomenon, individual or group, in order to establish its structure or behaviour. It is cross-sectional, because the phenomena being investigated are captured when they manifest themselves during a static moment of data collection, as stated by *(Polit and Hungler, 2003)*. Its purpose is to describe variables, and to analyse their incidence and interrelation at a given moment.

Population and Sample

The population is defined as the set of elements whose characteristics need to be known or investigated (Arias, ob.cit.). The population will be made up of patients between 7 and 13 years, 11 months and 29 days old, with attempted autolysis admitted to the emergency department of the Servicio Desconcentrado Hospital Universitario Pediátrico Dr. Agustín Zubillaga during the period January 2017 to June 2022, taking into account that it includes up to 13 years of age completely and not 14 years of age, since up to this age group is the age of hospitalisation in this hospital.

Now, for Hernández, Fernández, and Baptista, (2006) the sample is the group in which the study is conducted and is a set of units, a portion of the total, which represents the behaviour of the universe as a whole. However, in this case, the sampling is non-probabilistic, intentional, of the census type and will be made up of the patients mentioned previously and who meet the inclusion and exclusion criteria.

Inclusion Criteria

Patients with attempted autolysis admitted to the emergency department of the Servicio Desconcentrado Hospital Universitario Pediátrico Dr. Agustín Zubillaga during the period January 2017 to June 2022.

Patients of both sexes.

Patients between 7 and 13 years of age.

Exclusion Criteria

Patients admitted in a different time period and at a different age.

Procedure

A series of activities will be carried out in order to initiate the research and achieve the proposed objective, which are described below:

1. Request for permission to the governing body of the Servicio Desconcentrado Hospital Universitario Pediátrico Dr. Agustín Zubillaga, to carry out the study through correspondence prepared for this purpose (Annex A).

2. Request for permission from the Bioethics Committee of the Hospital Universitario Pediátrico Dr. Agustín Zubillaga (Annex B).

3. Collect the required data on the collection sheet (Annex C).

4. Preparation of the database with the use of Microsoft Excel spreadsheet. Tabulation of the data.

5. Analysis of data and their representation in tables and graphs.

6. Discussion.

7. Drawing up conclusions and recommendations.

Data Collection Technique and Instrument

In order to obtain the necessary information, it is very important to clearly define the collection techniques and instruments that will be used to obtain the data from reality applied to the situation to be studied, for its subsequent analysis. According to Arias (ob.cit.), data collection techniques are the different ways of obtaining information. In this research, a data collection form will be used as a secondary source. As for the instruments, the aforementioned author states that they constitute the materials used to collect the information. A data collection form was used, which is an instrument that allowed the recording and identification of the sources of information, as well as the collection of data that facilitated the recording, organisation and classification of the information (Robledo, 2010). The form was designed for the study and consists of four parts (Annex C):

1. Part I: Demographic data

2. Part II: Clinical features.

3. Part III: Risk factors

4. Part IV: Evolution

Data Processing and Analysis Techniques

For the processing and analysis of the data, SPSS for Windows version 25.0 was used. Descriptive statistical data were obtained, which, according to the objectives of the study, were processed, analysed and presented in statistical tables in absolute figures and percentages, comparing them in their discussion with various previous research studies and literature on the topic under study, in order to finally draw conclusions and recommendations.

CHAPTER IV

RESULTS

The will to live or not to live should be assessed at all levels of the life of the person at risk, and to be able to act, as far as possible, in stages before the crisis is triggered. In view of the above, the following results provide relevant information.

Table 1

Absolute and percentage age distribution of the sample.

Category	fa	%
7 to 9 years	3	9%
10 to 12 years	14	40%
13 and over	18	51%
Total	35	100%

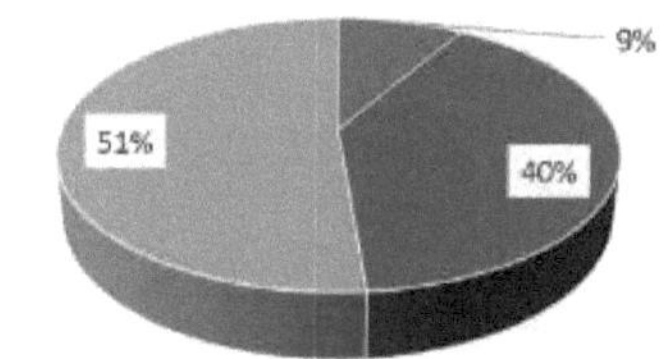

Graph 1 Age of the sample.

In the age group 13 years and older the results reached 51% while in the age group 10 to 12 years 40% and 7 to 9 years 9%.

Table 2

Absolute and percentage distribution of the sex of the sample.

SexofaX
Female   2263%
Male1337% Male1337% Male1337% Male1337% Male1337% Male1337% Male1337%
Male

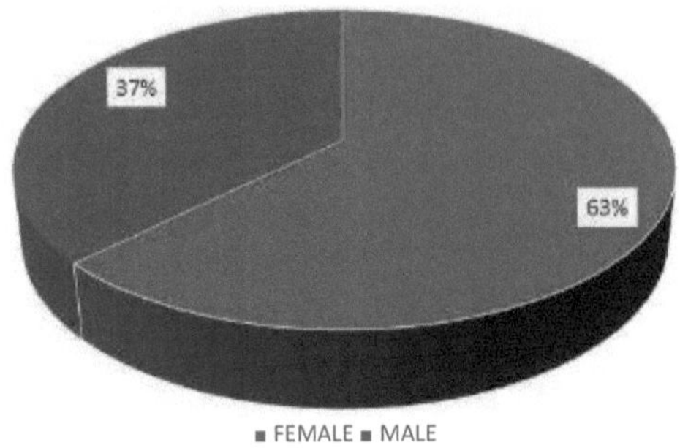

Figure 2 Sex of the sample.

The predominant sex in the sample was female (63%) and male (37%).

Absolute and percentage distribution of pathological antecedents.

Suffered from any illness	fa	%
Yes	6	17
No	29	83

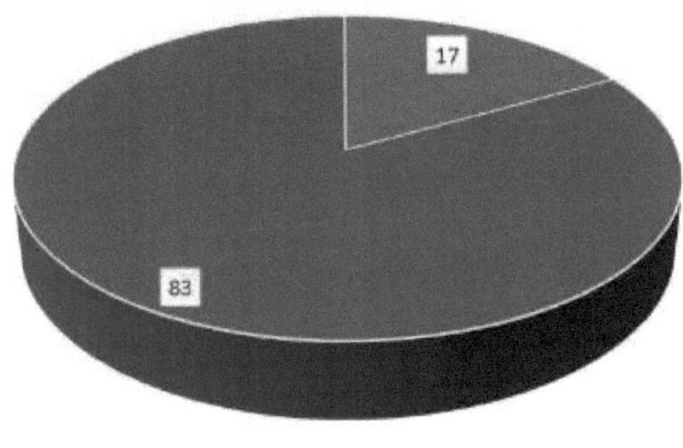

Graph 3 pathological history.

In 83% of the cases there was no disease and 17% had no underlying pathology.

Table 4

Absolute and percentage distribution of illness suffered.

ADHD	1	3%
Brain irritation	1	3%
Asthma	4	11%
Epilepsy	1	3%
total	7	20%

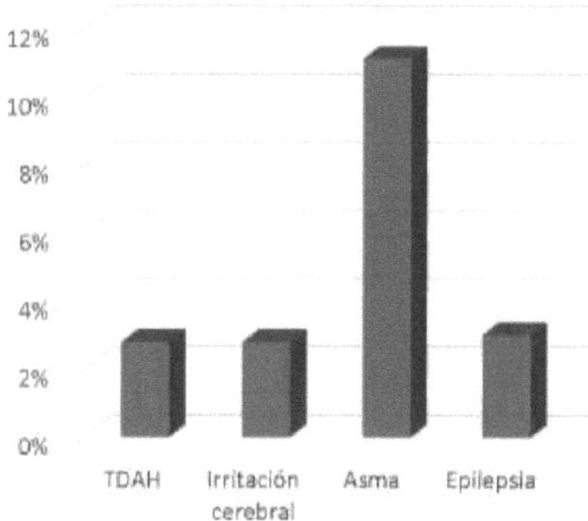

Figure 4 Illness from which you suffer.

Among the diseases they suffered from were asthma with 11%, brain irritation, epilepsy and ADHD in 3% of cases.

Table 5

Absolute and percentage distribution of psychiatric pathology.

Psychiatric	fa	%
Yes	1	3%
No	34	97%
Total	35	100

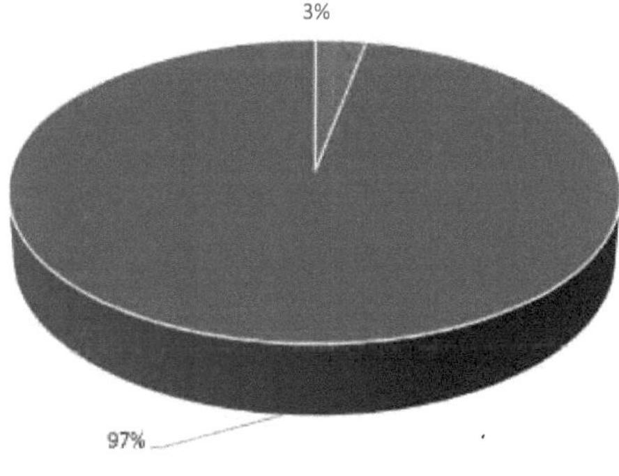

Graph 5 Psychiatric pathology.

Of the sample taken only 3% suffered from a psychiatric pathology and 97% did not suffer from psychiatric disorders.

Absolute and percentage distribution of medicine intake.

Take any medication	fa	%
Yes	5	14%
No	30	86%
Total	35	100%

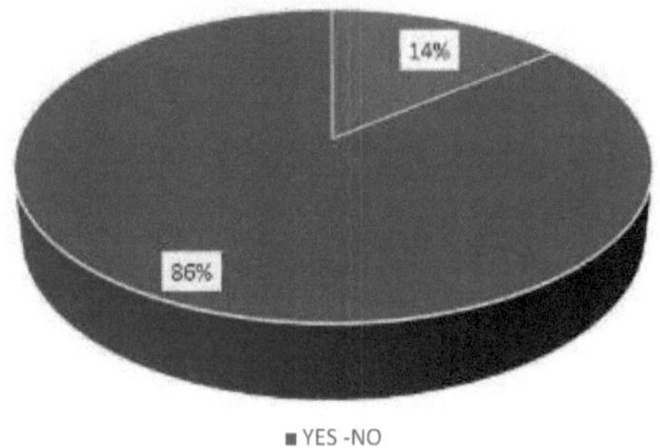

Figure 6 Medication intake.

Among the medication history, 86% did not take any medication and 14% did take medication.

Absolute and percentage distribution of medicines consumed.

Medicines	fa	%
Tegretol	1	3%
Trileptal	1	3%
Valproic acid	2	6%
Sertraline	1	1%

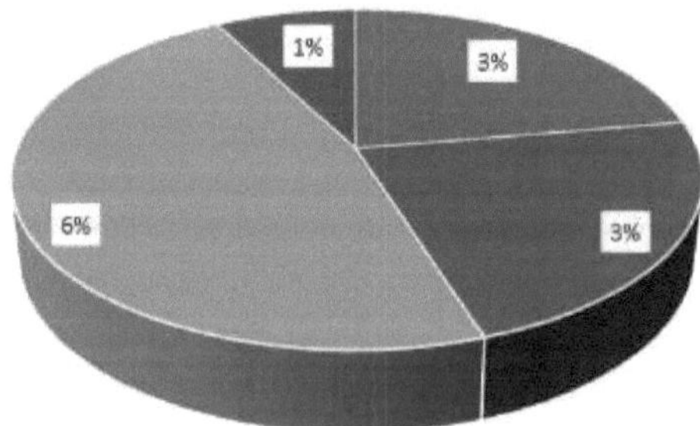

Graph 7 Medicines consumed.

Medications taken included valproic acid in 6% of cases, tegretol and trileptal in 3% and sertraline in 1% of cases.

Absolute and percentage distribution of substance use as a method of suicide.

Substance ingestion	fa	%
Yes	27	78%
No	8	22%
Total	35	100%

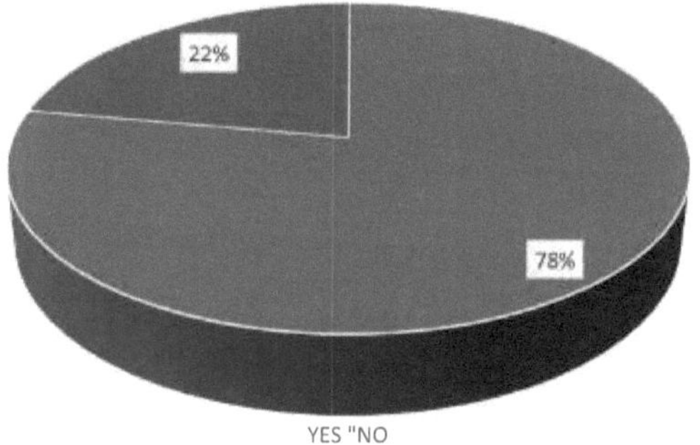

Figure 8 Substance ingestion as a method of suicide.

In 78% of the cases, some kind of substance was used as a method of suicide, while 22% did not.

Absolute and percentage distribution of the main medicines.

Medicines	fa	%
Alprazolam 1	2	6%
Bromazepam 10	1	3%
Carbamazepine 10	1	3%
Aspirin 100	1	3%
Valproic acid 15	1	3%
Alprazolam 15	1	3%
Cinnarizine 3	1	3%
Tegretol 5	1	3%
Cetirizine 7	1	3%
Phenobarbital 8	1	3%
Trileptal 8	1	3%
Amitraz	1	3%

Amoxicillin	1	3%
Atilan	1	3%
Champion	2	6%
Chlorine	1	3%
Herbicide	1	3%
Insecticide	1	3%
Nifedipine 8	3	8%
Not specified	2	6%
Omeprazole 100	1	3%
Paraquat	2	6%

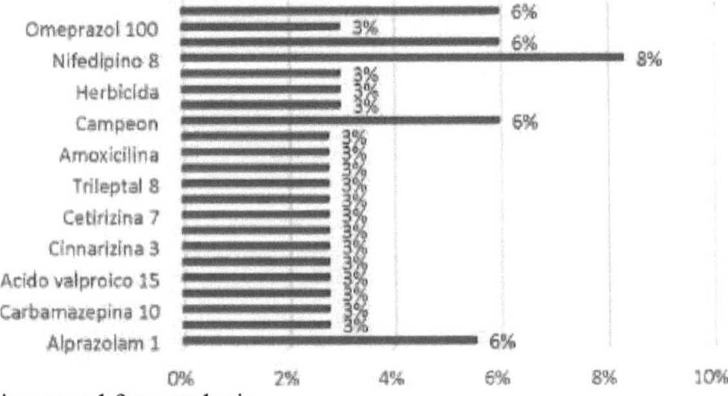

Figure 9 Medicines used for autolysis.

Nifedipine was used in 8% of cases, champion, Alprazolam and unspecified in 6%, in proportion of 3% other drugs (see table 9).

Table 10

Absolute and percentage distribution over substance injection.

Injection of substances	fa	%
Yes	1	3%
No	34	97%
Animal vitamin was injected		

3%

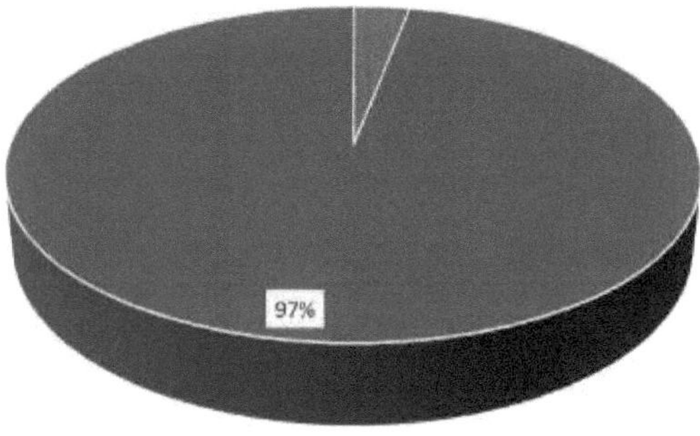

Figure 10 Injection of substances.

97% of cases did not use injecting substances and only 3% of cases were found to use injecting a substance.

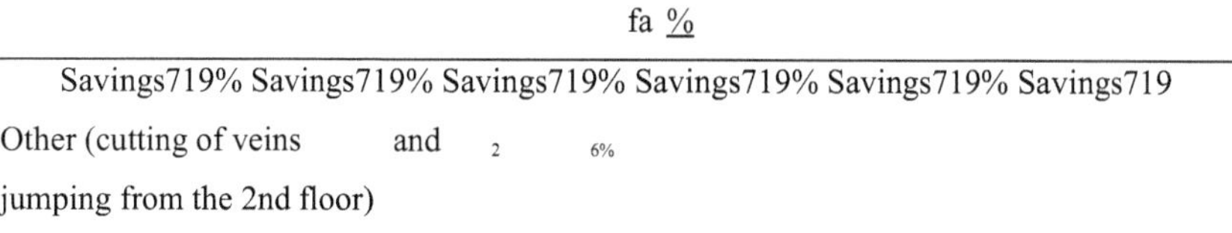

fa %

Savings719% Savings719% Savings719% Savings719% Savings719% Savings719

Other (cutting of veins and 2 6%

jumping from the 2nd floor)

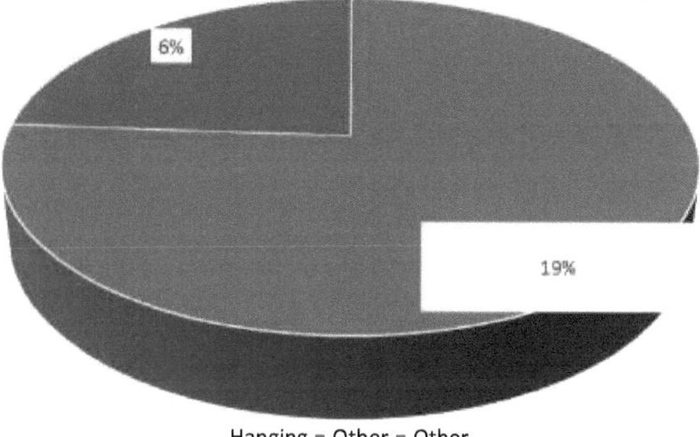

Figure 11 Methods used for autolysis.

The mechanism used for self-harm in 19 % was hanging. Six per cent used another mechanism, of which 3 per cent cut their veins and another 3 per cent threw themselves from a first floor.

Table 12

Absolute and percentage distribution place of suicide.

Place of suicide	fa	%

Your home	33	94%
Family	2	6%
Street	0	0%
School	0	0%
Other place	0	0%

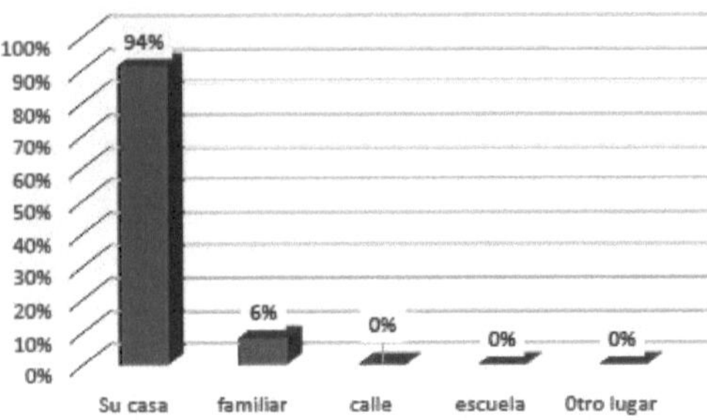

Figure 12 Place of suicide.

92% of the cases occurred at home, 8% at a relative's home.

Family history of suicide	fa	%	Who
No	29	83%	Aunt and uncles
Yes	6	17%	Parents
			Mother

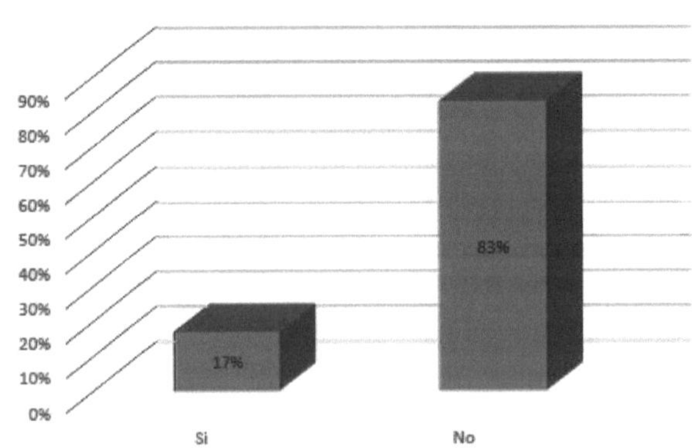

Figure 13 Family history of suicide.

83% of the cases had no family history, 17% had a history with fathers, uncles (maternal and paternal line) and other relatives.

	Death	fa	%
Yes		2	6%
No		33	94%
Total		35	100%

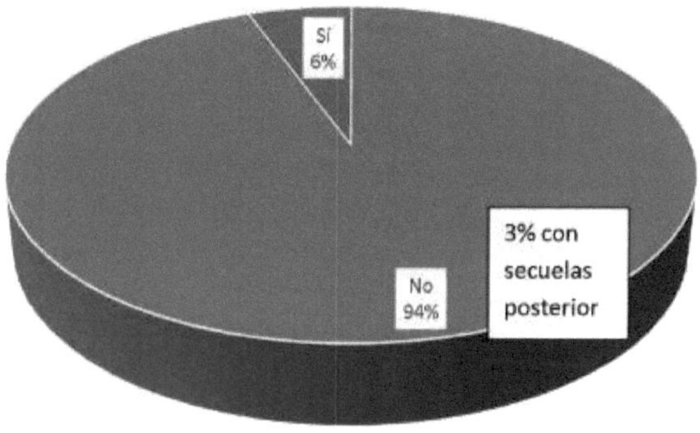

Graph 14 Death due to autolysis.

Although a minority of cases died (6%), of the remaining 94%, 3% were left with sequelae days after their attempt at self-harm.

Absolute and percentage distribution of the Graffar level.

	Graffar	fa	%
III		3	8%
IV		21	61%
V		11	31%
Total		35	100%

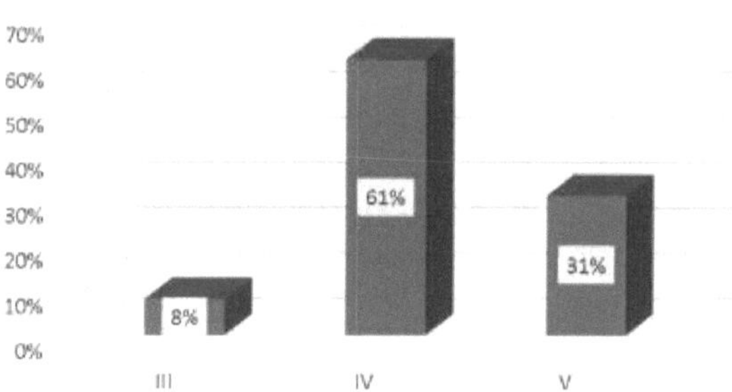

Graph 15 Graffar level.

On the Graffar scale, 61% were found to be in stratum IV, 31% in stratum V and 8% were in a grade III stratum according to their social classification.

Study	fa	%
Yes	32	91%
No	3	9%

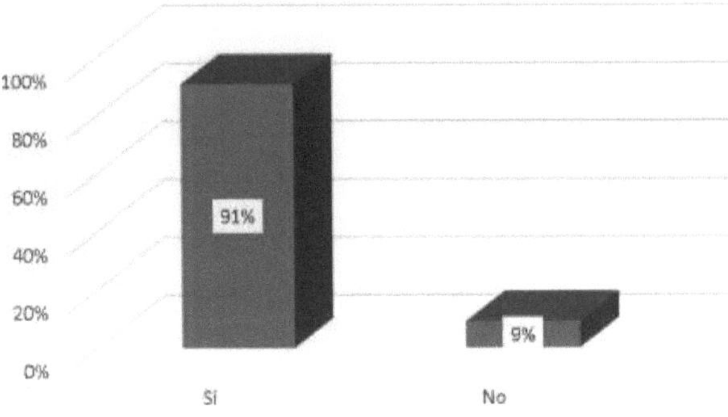

Graph 16 schooling.

On the level of schooling it was found that 91% studied and 9% did not.

Level	fa	%
Primary	8	23%
Secondary	27	77%
Illiterate	0	0%
Total	35	100%

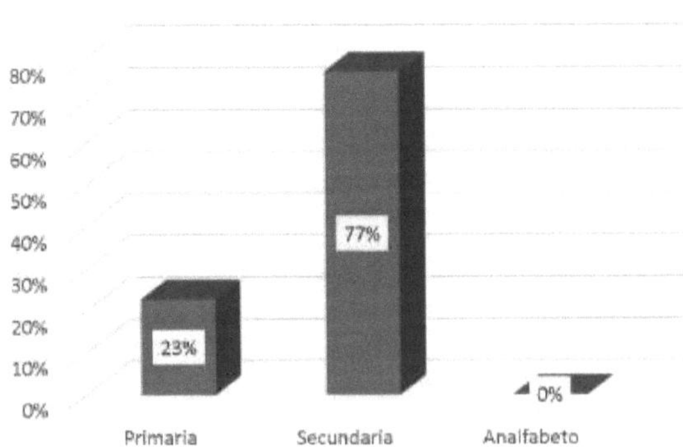

Graph 17 Educational level.

Of the educational level of the total sample, 77% had secondary schooling, 23% had primary schooling and no illiteracy was found.

Table 18

Absolute and percentage distribution of academic performance

Academic performance	fa	%
Good	9	26%
Regular	18	51%
Deficient	8	23%
Totals	35	100%

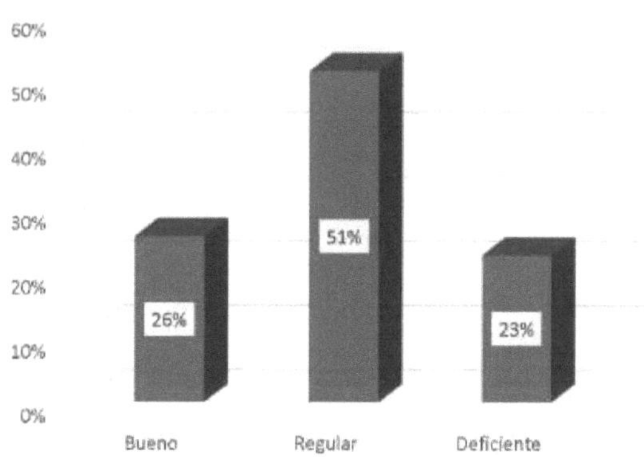

Graph 18 Academic performance.

Regarding academic performance 51% are fair, 26% are good and 23% are poor.

Absolute and percentage distribution of work.

Work	fa	%
No	35	100%
Yes	0	0%
Total	35	100%

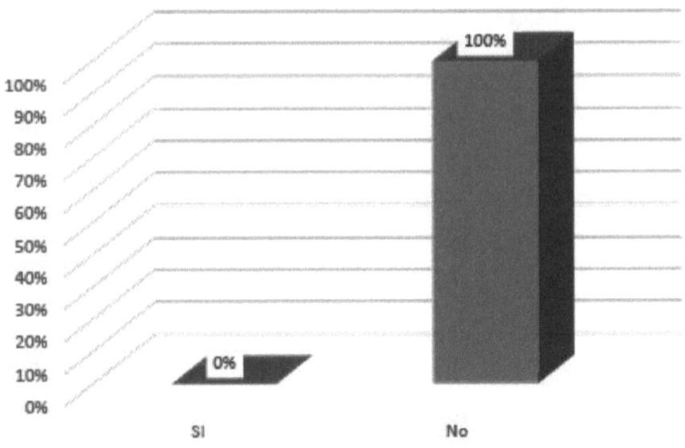

Graph 19

100% of the patients were not involved in work activities.

Absolute and percentage distribution of the number of family members.

Members	fa	%
3	4	11%
4	15	42%
5	8	23%
6	3	9%
7	2	6%
8	1	3%
12	2	6%
Total	35	100%

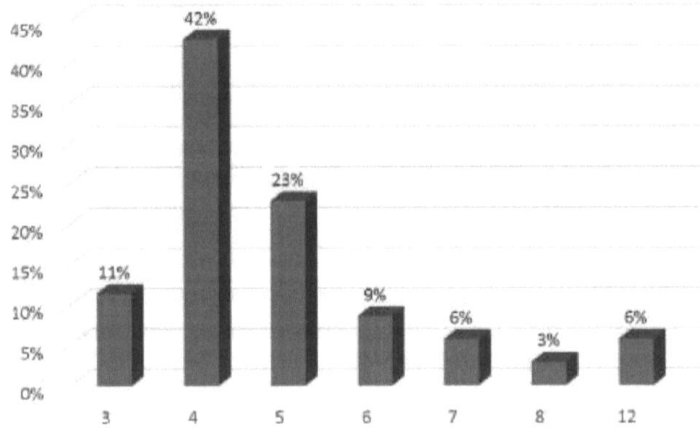

Figure 20 Number of family members.

The highest number of family members is 12 persons and represents 6% of the cases, families with 4 members 42%, those with 5 members 23%, 3 members 11%, 6 members 9%, 7 members 6% and 8 members 3%.

Relative with whom you live	fa	%
Parents and siblings	6	17%
Maternal grandmother, aunts, uncles and siblings	2	6%
Grandparents	1	3%
Mother, stepfather and brother	1	3%
Mother and siblings	13	39%
Father and brother	11	30%
Not specified	1	3%
Total	35	100%

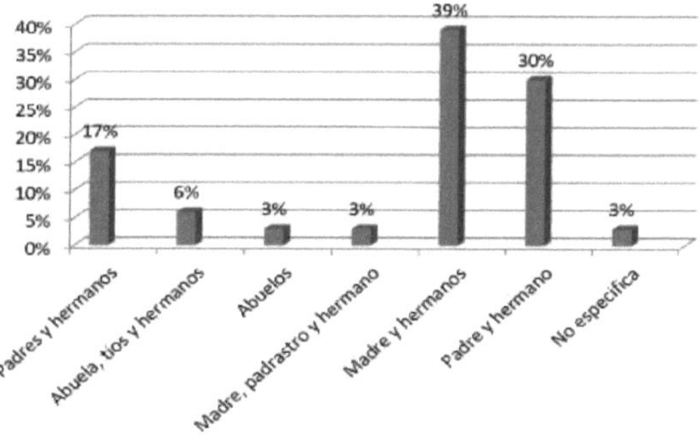

Graph 21 on who you live with.

39% of the study sample live with their mother and siblings, 30% with their father and siblings, 17% live with both parents and siblings, 3% live with their grandparents, step-mother and step-sibling or not specified.

Representative	fa	%
Mother	18	50%
Grandma	6	17%
Father	4	11%
Not specified	7	22%
Total	35	100%

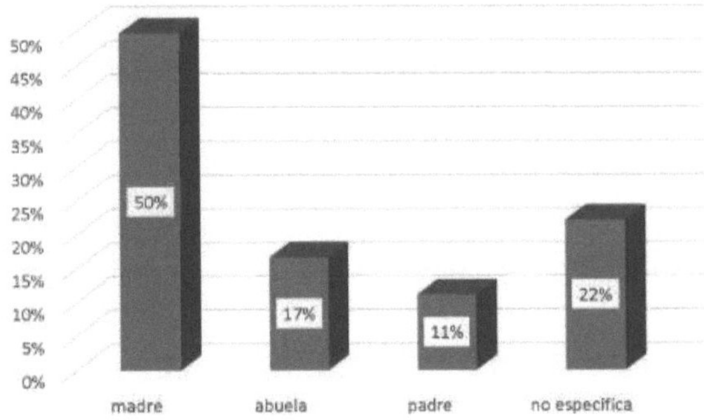

Figure 22

The majority is represented by their mother in 50% of the cases, 22% non-specific, 17% by their grandmother and by the father in 11% of the cases.

Absent parents	fa	%	Which
One	19	54%	
Who	19	54%	father
Both	6	17%	

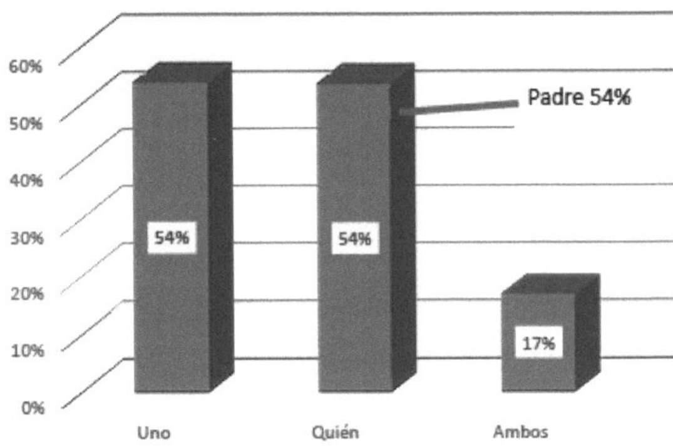

Figure 23 Absent parents.

Of the 54% of the sample, at least one parent was absent, 54% of the sample had an absent father figure, and 17% had both parents absent.

Table 24

Absence reason for absence in absolute and percentage distribution.

Reason for absence	fa	%
Abandonment	2	6%
Low resources	5	14%
Divorce due to violence	1	3%

Deceased and emigrated	3	8%
Migrated to Chile,	4	11%
Deprived of liberty	2	6%
Separation	8	22%
Unknown	1	3%

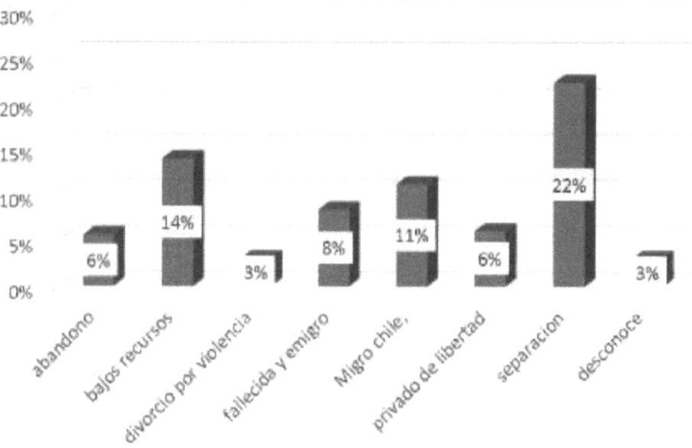

Graph 24 Reason for absence.

Of the causes of the absence of one or both parents, parental separation accounts for 22% of the cases, low income 14%, migration to Chile 11%, death or emigration 8%, abandonment and deprivation of liberty 6%, another variety of reasons are divorce due to violence, and unknown causes account for 3% of the cases.

Table 25

Absolute and percentage distribution on the type of Relationship with parents.

Relationship with parents	fa	%
Good	5	14%
Regular	4	11%
Mala	7	19%
It does not exist	12	33%
Total	28	78%

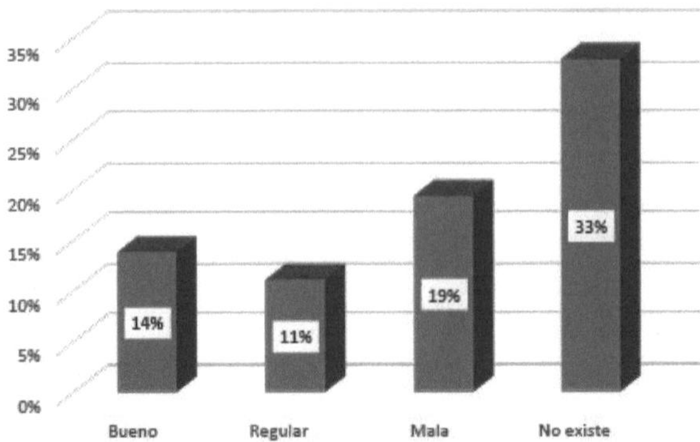

Graph 25 Relationship with parents.

The information does not reach 100% as there is an underreporting of data. The majority had no relationship with the parents, which represented 33% of the cases, 19% had a bad relationship with the parents, 14% had a good relationship and 11% had a regular relationship with the parents.

Table 26

Absolute and percentage distribution of attempts.

YES			NO		
	fa	%	fa	%	When
Has previous attempts at self-harm	10	28%	24		67%Average time in months
Warned of wanting to commit self-harm	13	36%	22	61%	3,125

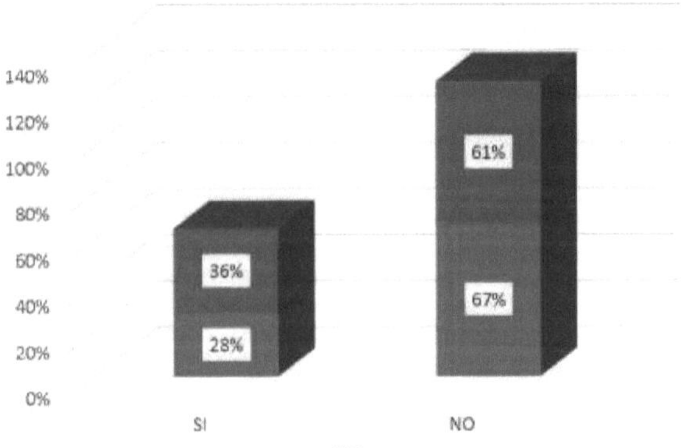

Graph 26 Attempted self-harm.

Regarding attempts at self-harm, 28% had attempted it before and 67% had not attempted it before. In relation to whether they had warned of wanting to commit self-harm, 36% had warned and 61% had not warned.

Table 27

Absolute and percentage distribution To whom I participate.

To whom I participate	fa	%
relatives	5	14%
mum	1	3%

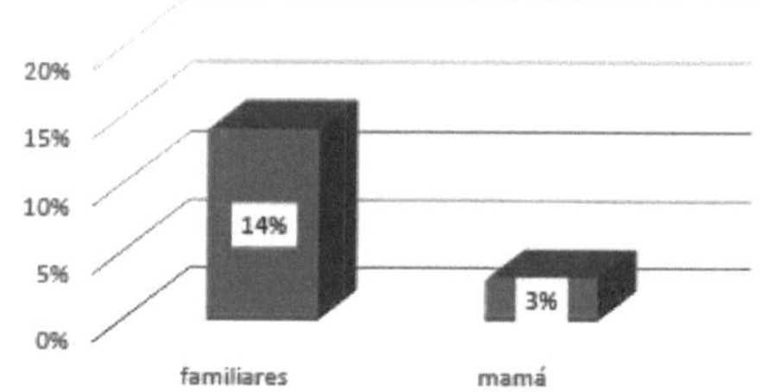

Graph 27 To whom did you share your intention of self-harm?

14% of the cases involved their relatives and 3% their mother directly. These were the data that were processed based on the information collected in the form.

Table 28

Absolute and percentage distribution of Reason for Attempt.

reason for the attempt	fa	%
Fight with family member	18	51%
Discussion with the mother	6	17%
Depression	3	9%
Mother punishes	3	9%
Feels in the way	2	6%
Bullying at school	1	3%
I hear voices	1	3%
By separation	1	3%
Doing poorly in studies	1	3%

It does not explain	1	3%

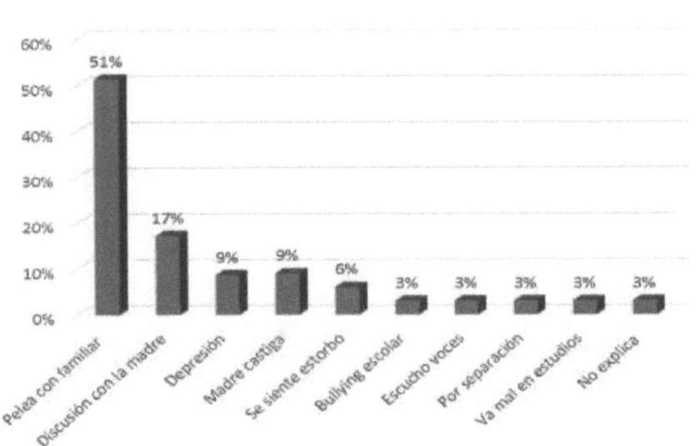

Graph 28 Reason for attempted self-harm.

In 51% of the cases the action is motivated by a fight with relatives, 17% by an argument with their mother, 9% by depression or punishment from their mother, 6% feel they are a nuisance, and the rest of the reasons such as bullying at school, hearing voices, separation or doing badly at school, others represent 3% of the cases.

Discussion of results

In this study, 51% of the population was aged 13 and over, and 63% of the female sex. Similar results were obtained in Loja and Zamora Chinchipe - Ecuador (2018), where they found that the most affected sex was male, aged between 12 and 17 years old.

Among those with a history of medication, 86% did not take any medication at all. Among those who did have a history of medication, they took valproic acid in 6% of cases, tegretol and trileptal in 3% and sertraline in 1% of cases. On the other hand, 83% of the cases did not suffer from any illnesses and among those who did have pathology were asthma with 11%, cerebral irritation, epilepsy and ADHD in 3% of the cases. Only 17% of the sample was found to have a pathology. These findings are different from those of Arencibia (2022) who found a high number of young patients with psychiatric problems and attempted self-harm.

On the other hand, 78% of the cases ingested some kind of substance, multiple medications were used, among the most common were Nifedipine in 8% of cases, champion, Alprazolam and unspecified in 6%, in proportion of 3% other medications (see table 9). Vega (2021) found that the majority of his sample attempted suicide due to drug intoxication. As for injections, only 3% used injections of substances and cutting of veins, in addition to throwing themselves from a first floor was a mechanism used, and 19% used hanging as a method. One of these mechanisms of self-harm was ratified in the study of Loja and Zamora Chinchipe (2018), as hanging was the most common mechanism used in Ecuador.

Ninety-one percent of the cases occurred at home, 9% at the home of a relative; at the socio-economic level, the most representative sample with 61% is found in the Graffar IV scale, in its social classification, taking into account that it is currently a very predominant stratum in our society. From the point of view of the level of schooling, it was found that 91% are studying and 9% are not. The educational level of the total sample was found to be 72% with a secondary school level, with a majority academic performance of 50% being regular. The highest number of family members is 16 persons in 44% of the cases and 5 persons in 22% of the cases.

39% of the sample under study live with their mother and siblings, 30% with their father and siblings. The majority is represented by their mother in 50% of the cases. Of the 53% of the sample at least one parent was absent. The causes for the absence of one or both parents were determined by the separation of the parents in up to 22% of the cases, low income 14%, migration to Chile 11%, death or emigration 8%, abandonment and deprivation of liberty 6%, and a variety of other reasons are divorce, violence, as well as unknown causes, which account for 3% of the cases. The majority have no relationship with their parents, who represent 33% of the cases.

Regarding attempts at self-harm, 28% had attempted it before and 67% had not attempted it before. In relation to whether they had warned their relatives about the intention to commit self-harm, 36% had warned them, 61% had not. In 51% of the cases, the action was motivated by a fight with relatives, 17% by an argument with their mother, 9% by depression or punishment from their mother, 6% felt they were a nuisance, and the rest of the reasons such as bullying at school, hearing voices, separation or doing badly at school, among others, represented 3% of the cases. It is worth noting that of the 100% of the sample, 6% died days after the attempt at self-harm and 3% had after-effects as a consequence of their actions.

CHAPTER V

CONCLUSIONS AND RECOMMENDATIONS
Conclusions

After analysing the data, the following conclusions can be drawn:

- The most common age group for attempted self-harm is around 13 years old and female.

- Among the medication history the majority did not take any medication at all, while among the percentage who did take valproic acid, tegretol and trileptal and sertraline were minimal.

- The majority of the cases did not suffer from any disease, while those who did have pathology were found to have asthma, brain irritation, epilepsy and ADHD.

- The majority of the sample ingested some type of substance, multiple medications were used; among the most common were Nifedipine, poisonous substance as champion, Alprazolam and others not specified.

- As for injections, only a small percentage used injections of substances and cutting of veins, as well as throwing oneself from a first floor and hanging, which were rarely used.

- Most of the cases occurred at home, a small percentage at a relative's home.

- At the socio-economic level, the sample is in the Graffar IV scale in most cases in their social classification.

- From the point of view of the level of schooling it was found that almost the totality of the sample studies. Most of them have a secondary school level, and their academic performance is mostly average.

- The highest number of family members is 16 persons in almost half of the sample of 5 persons in a smaller number of cases.

- The study sample is more likely to live with their mother and siblings, while the rest live with their father and siblings.

- Most are represented by their mother.

- These causes of absence of one or both parents are represented by separation with the highest frequency, followed by low income, migration, death, abandonment and deprivation of liberty, another variety of reasons are divorce due to violence, and unknown causes are also found in a lower percentage of cases.

- Most of them have no relationship with their parents.

- As for attempts at self-harm, most have not attempted it before without warning.

- Half of the cases the action is motivated by a fight with relatives, an argument with their mother, depression or punishment by their mother, they feel they are a nuisance, and the rest of the reasons such as bullying at school, hearing voices, separation or doing badly at school.

Recommendations

After that, the following can be recommended:

• Parents should be observant and vigilant of their children's attitudes and behavioural changes, so that when these occur they seek help immediately.

• Take preventive therapy and parenting education consultations for children and adolescents, especially in the pre-puberty and puberty stages.

• Encourage schools to provide counselling classes for children and adolescents in order to detect possible behaviours leading to suicide or suicide attempts.

• See a psychologist or psychiatrist if behavioural changes are observed, and normalise visits to these specialists.

• Remain vigilant of their children's activities, promoting and encouraging sports routines or recreational activities.

• Encourage the creation of support groups for children and adolescents in particularly difficult circumstances, both in schools and in other institutions.

- Insist that the records have more information on the psycho-emotional sphere of this type of patient.

BIBLIOGRAPHICAL REFERENCES

Arencibia 2022 attempted autolysis by intoxication in young Canarians: emergency department of the university hospital complex of the Canary Islands. Tenerife, Canary Islands

Argota N, Alvarez M, Camilo V, Sánchez Y, Barceló M. 2014 Behaviour of some risk factors for suicide attempts in adolescents. Rev. Med.

Arias, F. (2006). *El Proyecto de Investigación: Introducción a la metodología científica* (5th Ed.). Caracas: Editorial Episteme.

Arias, F. (2014). Introduction to Scientific Methodology: The Research Project. Mexico D. F., Mexico: Editorial Limusa S. A.

Asarnow JR, Hughes JL, Babeva KN, Sugar CA. *J2017* Cognitive-Behavioral Family Treatment for Suicide Attempt Prevention: A Randomized Controlled Trial.

Aucapiña Jenny. Factors associated with suicidal thoughts in adolescents of the Dora Beatriz Canelos Educational Unit. Final thesis report. Cuenca: Universidad de Cuenca, Facultad de ciencias médicas Escuela de enfermeria; 2019.

Constitution of the Bolivarian Republic of Venezuela (2009). Official Gazette No. 5.908 Extraordinary of 19 February 2009. Bolivarian Republic of Venezuela.

Daniel S, Mario V, Benjamin V, Esteban A, Rafaella D, Carolina S. Suicide attempt and risk factors in a sample of adolescents. Journal of Psychopathology and Clinical Psychology. 2017; 22(33-42).

Fonseca (2020) conducted a study entitled Assessment of suicidal behaviour in adolescents: a review of the Paykel Suicide Scale.

Hernández, S., Fernández, C and Baptista, P. (2006). *Research Methodology* (3rd edition). Madrid: Mc Graw Hill.

National Institute of Statistics and Census cited in Gerstner, (2018).

Kennebeck S, et al. Suicidal behavior in children and adolescents: Evaluation and management. https://www.uptodate.com/contents/search. Accessed March 23, 2021

The World Health Organisation (WHO 2020) suicidal behaviour.

Law on the Practice of Medicine (Amended 2011, December). Official Gazette No. 39823. Bolivarian Republic of Venezuela.

Ley Orgánica de Seguridad Social (2002). Bolivarian Republic of Venezuela.

Nixon K, Cloutier P, Jansson S. Nonsuicidal self-harm in youth: a population-based survey. Canadian Medical Association Journal. 2008; 178 (306-312).

Pan American Health Organization. Suicide prevention: a global imperative. Washington, DC. 2014.

Palella, S., and Martins, F. (2012). *Metodología De La Investigación Cuantitativa.* 3rd Ed.

Caracas: Edupel.

Polit, D., Hungler, B. (2003). Scientific *research* in health sciences. (6ª Ed). Mexico: McGraw- Hill Interamericana.

Robledo, C. (2010). *Data collection.* [Online document]. Available: https://investigar1.files.wordpress.com/2010/05/fichas-de-trabajo.pdf.

Tamayo y Tamayo, M. (2009). The Process of Scientific Research. Mexico, D. F., Mexico: Editorial Limusa.

Vega C., Esther (2021), "Defunciones por autolisis en el Centro de Investigación de Ciencias Forenses de la ciudad de Loja". Centro de Investigación de Ciencias Forenses de Loja-ecuador,

Villamar A. "Estudio retrospectivo del suicidio en el Instituto de Neurociencias 2011 - 2012". Guayaquil: Instituto de Neurociencias; 2015.

McKeown, R., Garrison, C., and Cuffe, S. (1998). Incidence and predictors of suicidal behaviour in a longitudinal sample of young adolescents. Journal of the American Academy of Child & Adolescent Psychiatry. Medline: https://www.jaacap.org/article/S0890-8567(09)63071-9/pdf.

ELMUNDO.es MADRID. Why does an 11-year-old child commit suicide? A website of Unidad Editorial UPDATED 21/10/2015. Disponible: https://www.elmundo.es/sociedad/2015/10/21/562699ac46163f44188b45d5.html [Consulta: 21/10/2015].

La Tercera: What do we know about child suicide? Trinidad Rojas. Available: https://www.latercera.com/paula/que-sabemos-sobre-el-suicidio-infantil/ [Accessed: 19/04/2022].

ANNEXES

Annex A

Authorisation request to the Hospital Director

UNIVERSIDAD CENTROCCIDENTAL "LISANDRO ALVARADO"

DEAN'S OFFICE OF HEALTH SCIENCES "DR PABLO ACOSTA ORTIZ".

POSTGRADUATE COURSE IN CHILDCARE AND PAEDIATRICS

Dr. Miriam Lucena

Director of HUPAZ

Present

Yours sincerely. I hereby inform you of my intention to develop a research project entitled: **FREQUENCY OF AUTOLYSIS ATTEMPT AND THE ASSOCIATED RISK FACTORS IN PATIENTS 7 TO 13 YEARS OF AGE WHO ENTER THE EMERGENCY OF THE UNIVERSITY HOSPITAL DISCONCENTRATED SERVICE PEDIATRIC PEDIATRIC DR. AGUSTÍN ZUBILLAGA DURING THE PERIOD FROM JANUARY 2017 TO JUNE 2022.** For this reason I request your authorisation to carry out this work.

For no other reason, I bid you a very cordial farewell.

you.

Yours faithfully.

Dr. Rafael Yépez

Paediatrics and Childcare Resident

Annex B

Application for Authorisation Bioethics Commission

UNIVERSIDAD CENTROCCIDENTAL "LISANDRO ALVARADO" DECANATO DE CIENCIAS DE LA SALUD "DR PABLO ACOSTA ORTIZ" POSTGRADO DE PUERICULTURA Y PEDIATRÍA . Dr. Julio Ochoa Bioethics Committee

Your Office

I would like to extend my warmest greetings and request your authorisation to carry out the study entitled: **FREQUENCY OF AUTOLYSIS ATTEMPTIONS AND THE ASSOCIATED RISK FACTORS IN PATIENTS AGED 7 TO 13 YEARS OF AGE ENTERING THE EMERGENCY DEPARTMENT OF THE UNIVERSITY HOSPITAL UNIVERSITY PAEDIATRIC DR. AGUSTÍN ZUBILLAGA DURING THE PERIOD FROM JANUARY 2017 TO JUNE 2022.** The data obtained will be handled with total confidentiality and for academic use only. It is worth noting that we do not intend to make a value judgement on the results obtained. If they are of interest to you, we will be happy to make them available to you at any time.

Thanking you in advance for your good offices in this regard,

Yours faithfully,

___

Dr. Rafael Yépez

Paediatrics and Childcare Resident

Annex C

LISANDRO ALVARADO" CENTRAL WESTERN UNIVERSITY

DEAN'S OFFICE OF HEALTH SCIENCES "DR PABLO ACOSTA ORTIZ"

POSTGRADUATE COURSE IN CHILDCARE AND PAEDIATRICS

FREQUENCY OF ATTEMPTED SELF-HARM AND

ASSOCIATED RISK FACTORS

IN PATIENTS AGED

7 TO 13 YEARS

ADMITTED TO THE EMERGENCY DEPARTMENT OF THE

DECONCENTRATED SERVICE OF THE

UNIVERSITY PAEDIATRIC

HOSPITAL DR. "AGUSTÍN ZUBILLAGA"

DURING THE PERIOD JANUARY 2017 TO JUNE 2022.

DATA COLLECTION INSTRUMENT

I. SOCIO-DEMOGRAPHIC DATA

1. Gender: male ___ female ___

2. Age: ___ years

II. CLINICAL DATA

3. Do you take any medication: Yes: ___ No: ___ Which one:

4. Do you have any underlying pathology?

a) Medical or Organic: Which

b) Psychiatric: Which

5. Mechanism of the Autolysis Attempt:

a) Ingestion of substance: O Which

b) Substance injection: Q Which

c) Hanging: □

d) Other: Q Which

6. Place where the attempted self-harm occurred:

a) Your home: ___ Family member's home: ___

b) Other person's house: ___ Which

c) In the street: ___ At school:

d) Elsewhere: Which

7. Family history of suicide: YES: ___ NO: ___ Who

8. Died as a result of the attempted self-harm: Yes ___ No ___

9. He was left with some after-effects of the attempted self-harm:

Yes ___ No ___ Which

III. RISK FACTORS

10. Graffar

     11. Student: Yes ___ No ___ Primary ___ Secondary ___ Illiterate ___

     Academic Performance: Good ___ Fair ___ Poor ___ Average ___ Poor

12. Do you work: Yes___ No___ Where and in what job?

13. Number of household members: ___ persons

14. With whom he lives:

Who is your representative:

15. Absent parents: Yes ___ No ___ One ___ Who

Both ___ Reason for absence

Relationship with parents: Good ___ Fair ___ Poor ___ Nonexistent

16. Do you play sports: Yes ___ No ___ Which one?

17. He previously warned of wanting to commit attempted self-harm:

Yes ___ No ___ To whom

18. Previous attempts at self-injury: Yes ___ No ___ When

19.

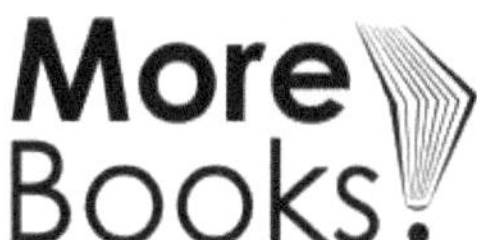

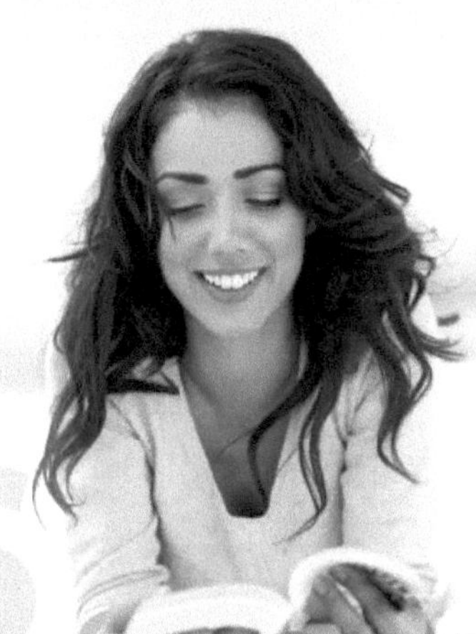

I want morebooks!

Buy your books fast and straightforward online - at one of world's fastest growing online book stores! Environmentally sound due to Print-on-Demand technologies.

Buy your books online at
www.morebooks.shop

Kaufen Sie Ihre Bücher schnell und unkompliziert online – auf einer der am schnellsten wachsenden Buchhandelsplattformen weltweit! Dank Print-On-Demand umwelt- und ressourcenschonend produzi ert.

Bücher schneller online kaufen
www.morebooks.shop

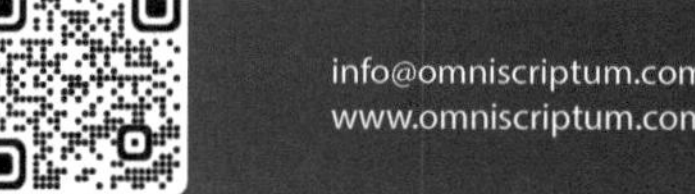

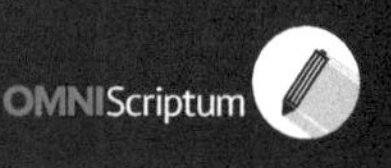